A NEW WAY OF CONSIDERING PLANTS

59 Easy and Tasty Plant-Based
Cookbook for Experts and Beginners
to Take Care Of Your Body and Soul

GREEN KITCHEN

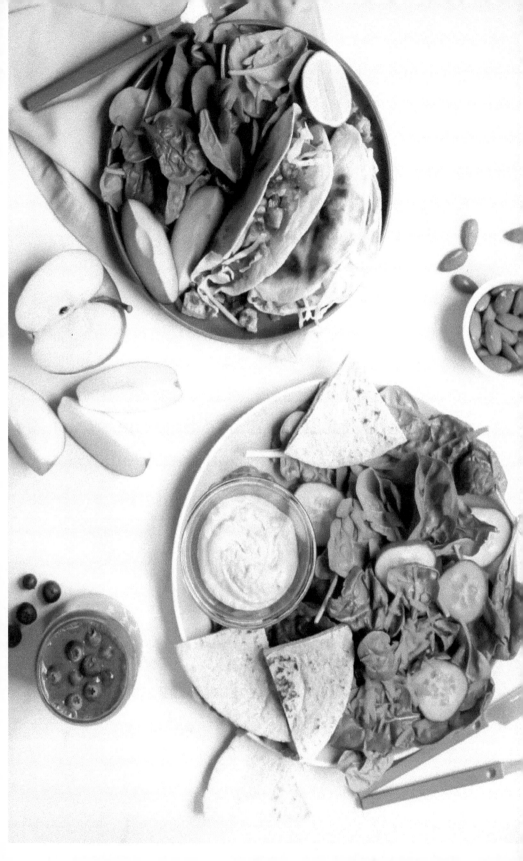

Table of Contents

INTRODUCTION

Eating healthy cannot be overemphasized in a world where fast food and junk food is always available. We all know that we could and should be eating healthier but there are so many diets being advertised that it's hard to know what's best for you.

We're always reading about how processed foods are bad for your body. You may have also been advised repeatedly to avoid foods high in preservatives; however, no one likes to eat bland food or spend their time reading labels. This book will teach you how to find nutritious, delicious foods that will keep you satisfied while improving your health.

BENEFITS OF A BALANCED DIET

Before we dive into talking about the recipes and foods you need for a balanced diet, let's discuss a little more on the need for eating balanced diet regularly.

- IMPROVED MEMORY: I know what you are thinking. "Are you being serious right now? If I just eat a few vegetables, I can be like Einstein?" Yes! You may not be as smart as Einstein, but healthy nutrients like Vitamins D, E, and C will help improve brain functionality.

- PREVENTS CANCER: According to medical experts, eating food that contains antioxidant can help protect cells from damage, thereby leading to a reduction in the risk of getting cancer. Cancer can also be treated at its early stage with healthy food.

- EMOTIONAL STABILITY: I know what you are thinking again. "Do you mean that if I'm going through a heartbreak and I eat some healthy food, I will be better?"

Yeah! It's not quite as straightforward as that, but healthy meals help improve your moods and balance your emotions. Scientists and researchers in 2016 found out that meals with a high glycemic load (high in carbohydrates) can trigger symptoms of depression and fatigue. Vegetables and fruits have a lower glycemic load and will help keep your blood sugar balanced.

- WEIGHT LOSS: Being overweight or obese can lead to other complicated illnesses like heart diseases, loss of bone density, and some types of cancer. Maintaining a healthful diet free from processed foods can help you stay at a healthy weight without resorting to fad diets.

- STRONG BONES AND TEETH: For healthy bones and teeth, a diet rich in calcium and magnesium is important. Maintaining bone integrity can reduce the risk of developing bone conditions later in life, such as osteoporosis.

Here are some foods that are rich in calcium:

- Low-fat dairy products
- Cabbage
- Legumes
- Broccoli
- Cauliflower
- Tofu

Now you know the awesome benefits of a healthy balanced diet, I'm sure you are on the edge of your seat waiting to see the healthy and easy-to-make meals planned out for you. Be sure to try them out and begin eating healthier today.
Enjoy!

BREAKFAST

Morning Nutty Oatmeal Muffins

Ready in about: 30 minutes

Servings: 18

Per serving: Calories: 192; Fat: 6g; Carbs: 30.5g; Protein: 5.6g

Ingredients

- 3 cups rolled oats
- 1 cup shredded coconut, unsweetened
- 3/2 teaspoons baking powder
- 1/2 teaspoon salt
- 1/2 teaspoon vanilla extract
- 1/2 teaspoon coconut extract
- 1/2 teaspoon grated nutmeg
- 1 teaspoon cardamom
- 3/2 cups coconut milk
- 1/6 cup canned pumpkin
- 1/8 cup agave syrup
- 1/8 cup golden raisins
- 1/8 cup pecans, chopped

Directions

1. Begin by preheating your oven to 360 degrees F. Spritz a muffin tin with nonstick cooking oil.
2. In a mixing bowl, thoroughly combine all the ingredients, except for the raisins and pecans.

3. Fold in the raisins and pecans and scrape the batter into the prepared muffin tin.
4. Bake your muffins for about 25 minutes or until the top is set.
5. Bon appétit!

Everyday Oats with Coconut and Strawberries

Ready in about: 15 minutes

Servings: 4

Per serving: Calories: 457; Fat: 14.4g; Carbs: 66.3g; Protein: 17.3g

Ingredients

- 1 tablespoon coconut oil
- 2 cups rolled oats
- A pinch of flaky sea salt
- 1/4 teaspoon grated nutmeg
- 1/2 teaspoon cardamom
- 2 tablespoons coconut sugar
- 2 cups coconut milk, sweetened
- 2 cups water
- 4 tablespoons coconut flakes
- 8 tablespoons fresh strawberries

Directions

1. In a saucepan, melt the coconut oil over a moderate flame. Then, toast the oats for about 3 minutes, stirring continuously.
2. Add in the salt, nutmeg, cardamom, coconut sugar, milk, and water; continue to cook for 12 minutes more or until cooked through.

3. Spoon the mixture into serving bowls; top with coconut flakes and fresh strawberries.
4. Bon appétit!

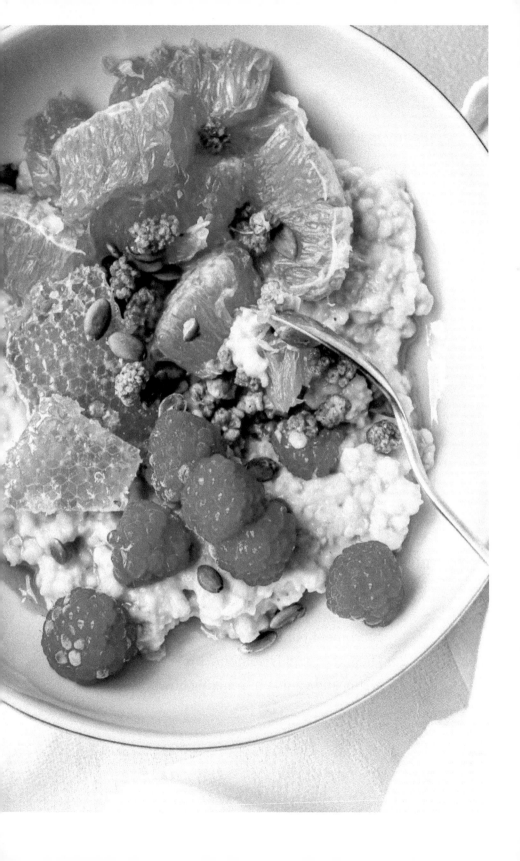

The Best Chocolate Granola Ever

Ready in about: 1 hour

Servings: 20

Per serving: Calories: 428; Fat: 23.4g; Carbs: 46.4g; Protein: 11.3g

Ingredients
- 1 cup coconut oil
- 1 cup agave syrup
- 2 teaspoons vanilla paste
- 6 cups rolled oats
- 1 cup hazelnuts, chopped
- 1 cup pumpkin seeds
- 1 teaspoon ground cardamom
- 2 teaspoons ground cinnamon
- 1/2 teaspoon ground cloves
- 2 teaspoons Himalayan salt
- 1 cup dark chocolate, cut into chunks

Directions
1. Begin by preheating your oven to 260 degrees F; line two rimmed baking sheets with a piece of parchment paper.
2. Then, thoroughly combine the coconut oil, agave syrup, and vanilla in a mixing bowl.

3. Gradually add in the oats, hazelnuts, pumpkin seeds, and spices; toss to coat well. Spread the mixture out onto the prepared baking sheets.
4. Bake in the middle of the oven, stirring halfway through the cooking time, for about 1 hour or until golden brown.
5. Stir in the dark chocolate and let your granola cool completely before storing. Store in an airtight container.
6. Bon appétit!

English Muffins with Tofu

Ready in about: 15 minutes

Servings: 8

Per serving: Calories: 452; Fat: 24.3g; Carbs: 38g; Protein: 25.6g

Ingredients

- 4 tablespoons olive oil
- 32 ounces extra-firm tofu
- 2 tablespoons nutritional yeast
- 1/2 teaspoon turmeric powder
- 4 handfuls fresh kale, chopped
- Kosher salt and ground black pepper, to taste
- 8 English muffins, cut in half
- 8 tablespoons ketchup
- 8 slices vegan cheese

Directions

1. Heat the olive oil in a frying skillet over medium heat. When it's hot, add the tofu and sauté for 8 minutes, occasionally stirring to promote even cooking.
2. Add in the nutritional yeast, turmeric, and kale, and continue sautéing for an additional 2 minutes or until the kale wilts. Season with salt and pepper to taste.
3. Meanwhile, toast the English muffins until crisp.

4. To assemble the sandwiches, spread the bottom halves of the English muffins with ketchup; top them with the tofu mixture and vegan cheese; place the bun topper on, close the sandwiches and serve warm.
5. Bon appétit!

Apple and Honey Toast

Ready in about: 5 minutes

Servings: 8

Per serving: Calories: 212 Cal Fat: 7 g Carbs: 35 g Protein: 4 g Fiber: 5.5 g

Ingredients:
- ½ of a small apple, cored, sliced
- 1 slice of whole-grain bread, toasted
- 1 tablespoon honey
- 2 tablespoons hummus
- 1/8 teaspoon cinnamon

Directions:
1. Spread hummus on one side of the toast, top with apple slices and then drizzle with honey.
2. Sprinkle cinnamon on it and then serve straight away.

Avocado Toast with Herbs and Peas

Ready in about: 10 minutes

Servings: 8

Per serving: Calories: 250 Cal Fat: 12 g Carbs: 22 g Protein: 7 g Fiber: 9 g

Ingredients:

- 1 of a medium avocado, peeled, pitted, mashed
- 12 slices of radish
- 4 tablespoons baby peas
- ½ teaspoon ground black pepper
- 2 teaspoons chopped basil
- ½ teaspoon salt
- 1 lemon, juiced
- 2 slices of bread, whole-grain, toasted

Directions:

1. Spread mashed avocado on one side of the toast and then top with peas, pressing them into the avocado.
2. Layer the toast with radish slices, season with salt and black pepper, sprinkle with basil, and drizzle with lemon juice.
3. Serve straight away.
4. Bon Appétit

Orange Butter Crepes

Ready in about: 5-15 minutes

Servings: 8

Per serving: Calories 379 Fats 35. 6g Carbs 14. 8g Protein 5. 6g

Ingredients:
- 2 tbsps flax seed powder + 6 tbsps water
- 1 tsp vanilla extract
- 1 tsp pure date sugar
- ¼ tsp salt
- 2 cups almond flour
- 1½ cups oat milk
- ½ cup melted plant butter
- 3 tbsps fresh orange juice
- 3 tbsps plant butter for frying

Directions:
1. In a medium bowl, mix the flax seed powder with 1 cup water and allow thickening for 5 minutes to make the flax egg. Whisk in the vanilla, date sugar, and salt.
2. Pour in a quarter cup of almond flour and whisk, then a quarter cup of oat milk, and mix until no lumps remain. Repeat the mixing process with the remaining almond flour and almond milk in the same quantities until exhausted.

3. Mix in the plant butter, orange juice, and half of the water until the mixture is runny like that of pancakes. Add the remaining water until the mixture is lighter. Brush a large nonstick skillet with some butter and place over medium heat to melt.

4. Pour 1 tablespoon of the batter into the pan and swirl the skillet quickly and all around to coat the pan with the batter. Cook until the batter is dry and golden brown beneath, about 30 seconds.

5. Use a spatula to carefully flip the crepe and cook the other side until golden brown too. Fold the crepe onto a plate and set it aside. Repeat making more crepes with the remaining batter until exhausted. Drizzle some maple syrup on the crepes and serve.

Irish Brown Bread

Ready in about: 5-15 minutes

Servings: 8

Per serving: Calories 963 Fats 44. 4g Carbs 125. 1g Protein 22. 1g

Ingredients:
- 8 cups whole-wheat flour
- ½ tsp salt
- 1 cup rolled oats
- 2 tsps baking soda
- 3 cups coconut milk, thick
- 4 tbsps pure maple syrup

Directions:
1. Preheat the oven to 400 F.
2. In a bowl, mix flour, salt, oats, and baking soda. Add in coconut milk, maple syrup, and whisk until dough forms. Dust your hands with some flour and knead the dough into a ball. Shape the dough into a circle and place it on a baking sheet.
3. Cut a deep cross on the dough and bake in the oven for 15 minutes at 450 F. Then, reduce the temperature to 400 F and bake further for 20 to 25 minutes or until a hollow sound is made when the bottom of the bread is tapped. Slice and serve.

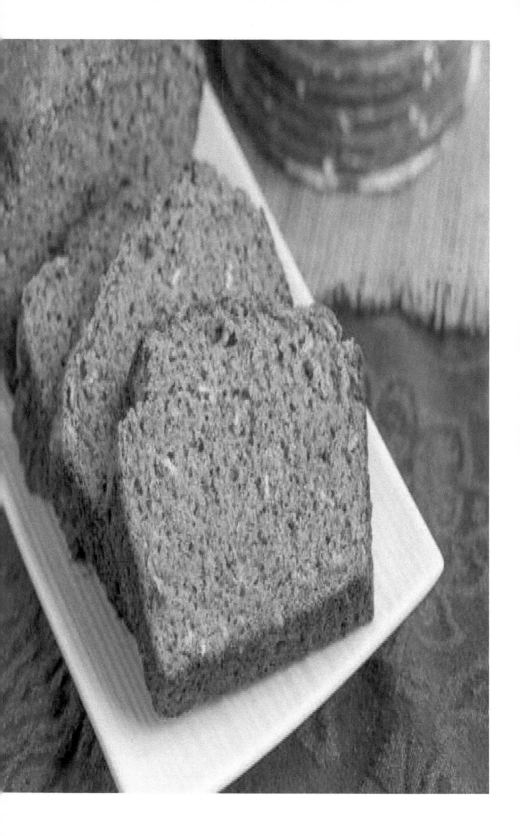

Almond & Raisin Granola

Ready in about: 20 minutes

Servings: 16

Ingredients

- 11 cups old-fashioned oats
- 3 cups chopped walnuts
- 1 cup shelled sunflower seeds
- 2 cups golden raisins
- 2 cups shaved almonds
- 2 cups pure maple syrup
- 1 tsp ground cinnamon
- ½ tsp ground allspice
- A pinch of salt

Directions

1. Preheat oven to 325 F. In a baking dish, place the oats, walnuts, and sunflower seeds. Bake for 10 minutes. Lower the heat from the oven to 300 F. Stir in the raisins, almonds, maple syrup, cinnamon, allspice, and salt. Bake for an additional 15 minutes. Allow cooling before serving.

Sweet Orange Crepes

Ready in about: 30 minutes

Servings: 8

Ingredients

- 4 tbsps flax seed powder
- 2 tsps vanilla extract
- 2 tsps pure date sugar
- ½ tsp salt
- 4 cups almond flour
- 3 cups oat milk
- 3 cups melted plant butter
- 6 tbsps fresh orange juice
- 6 tbsps plant butter for frying

Directions

1. In a medium bowl, mix the flax seed powder with 6 tbsps water and allow thickening for 5 minutes to make the vegan "flax egg." Whisk in the vanilla, date sugar, and salt.

2. Pour in a quarter cup of almond flour and whisk, then a quarter cup of oat milk, and mix until no lumps remain. Repeat the mixing process with the remaining almond flour and almond milk in the same quantities until exhausted.

3. Mix in the plant butter, orange juice, and half of the water until the mixture is runny like pancakes. Add the remaining water until the mixture is lighter. Brush a nonstick skillet with some butter and place over medium heat to melt.

4. Pour 1 tablespoon of the batter into the pan and swirl the skillet quickly and all around to coat the pan with the batter. Cook until the batter is dry and golden brown beneath, about 30 seconds.

5. Use a spatula to flip the crepe and cook the other side until golden brown too. Fold the crepe onto a plate and set it aside. Repeat making more crepes with the remaining batter until exhausted. Drizzle some maple syrup on the crepes and serve.

Simple Apple Muffins

Ready in about: 40 minutes

Servings: 8

Ingredients

For the muffins:

- 2 flax seed powder + 6 tbsps water

- 3 cups whole-wheat flour
- 2 cups pure date sugar
- 4 tsps baking powder
- ½ tsp salt
- 2 tsps cinnamon powder
- 2/3 cup melted plant butter
- 2/3 cup flax milk
- 4 apples, chopped

For topping:

- 2/3 cup whole-wheat flour

- 1 cup pure date sugar
- 1 cup cold plant butter, cubed
- 3 tsps cinnamon powder

Directions

1. Preheat oven to 400 F and grease 6 muffin cups with cooking spray. In a bowl, mix the flax seed

powder with water and allow thickening for 5 minutes to make the vegan "flax egg."

2. In a bowl, mix flour, date sugar, baking powder, salt, and cinnamon powder. Whisk in the butter, vegan "flax egg," flax milk, and fold in the apples. Fill the muffin cups two-thirds way up with the batter.

3. In a bowl, mix remaining flour, date sugar, cold butter, and cinnamon powder. Sprinkle the mixture on the muffin batter. Bake for 20 minutes. Remove the muffins onto a wire rack, allow cooling, and serve.

Blueberry Muesli Breakfast

Ready in about: 10 minutes

Servings: 10

Ingredients

- 4 cups spelt flakes
- 4 cups puffed cereal
- ½ cup sunflower seeds
- ½ cup almonds
- ½ cup raisins
- ½ cup dried cranberries
- ½ cup chopped dried figs
- ½ cup shredded coconut
- ½ cup non-dairy chocolate chips
- 6 tsps ground cinnamon
- 1 cup coconut milk
- 1 cup blueberries

Directions

1. In a bowl, combine the spelt flakes, puffed cereal, sunflower seeds, almonds, raisins, cranberries, figs, coconut, chocolate chips, and cinnamon. Toss to mix well. Pour in the coconut milk. Let sit for 1 hour and serve topped with blueberries.

2. Enjoy!

LUNCH

Country Cornbread with Spinach

Ready in about: 50 minutes

Servings: 16

Per serving: Calories: 282; Fat: 15.4g; Carbs: 30g; Protein: 4.6g

Ingredients

- 2 tablespoons flaxseed meal
- 2 cups all-purpose flour
- 2 cups yellow cornmeal
- 1 teaspoon baking soda
- 1 teaspoon baking powder
- 2 teaspoons kosher salt
- 2 teaspoons brown sugar
- A pinch of grated nutmeg
- 5/2 cups oat milk, unsweetened
- 2 teaspoons white vinegar
- 1 cup olive oil
- 4 cups spinach, torn into pieces

Directions

1. Start by preheating your oven to 420 degrees F. Now, spritz a baking pan with a nonstick cooking spray.
2. To make the flax eggs, mix flaxseed meal with 3 tablespoons of water. Stir and let it sit for about 15 minutes.

3. In a mixing bowl, thoroughly combine the flour, cornmeal, baking soda, baking powder, salt, sugar, and grated nutmeg.
4. Gradually add in the flax egg, oat milk, vinegar, and olive oil, constantly whisking to avoid lumps. Afterwards, fold in the spinach.
5. Scrape the batter into the prepared baking pan. Bake your cornbread for about 25 minutes or until a tester inserted in the middle comes out dry and clean.
6. Let it stand for about 10 minutes before slicing and serving. Bon appétit!

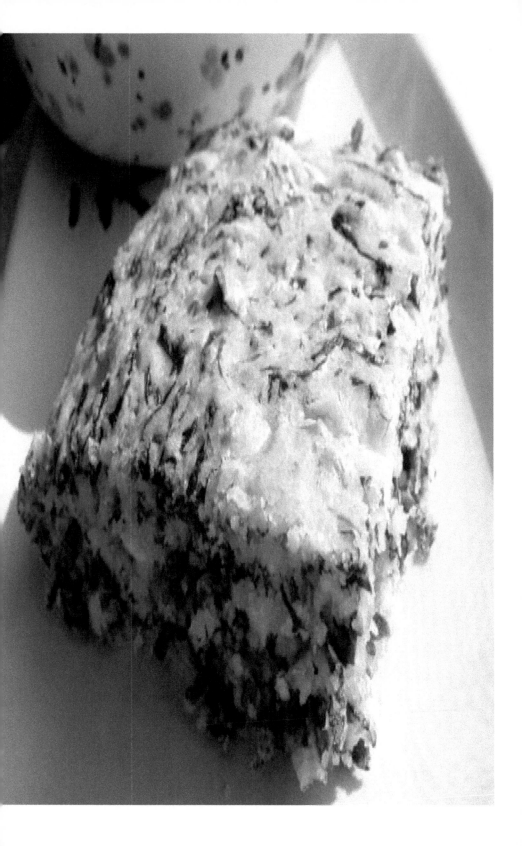

Millet Porridge with Sultanas

Ready in about: 25 minutes

Servings: 6

Per serving: Calories: 353; Fat: 5.5g; Carbs: 65.2g; Protein: 9.8g

Ingredients

- 2 cups water
- 2 cups coconut milk
- 2 cups millet, rinsed
- 1/2 teaspoon grated nutmeg
- 1/2 teaspoons ground cinnamon
- 2 teaspoons vanilla paste
- 1/2 teaspoon kosher salt
- 4 tablespoons agave syrup
- 8 tablespoons sultana raisins

Directions

1. Place the water, milk, millet, nutmeg, cinnamon, vanilla, and salt in a saucepan; bring to a boil.
2. Turn the heat to a simmer and let it cook for about 20 minutes; fluff the millet with a fork and spoon into individual bowls.
3. Serve with agave syrup and sultanas. Bon appétit!

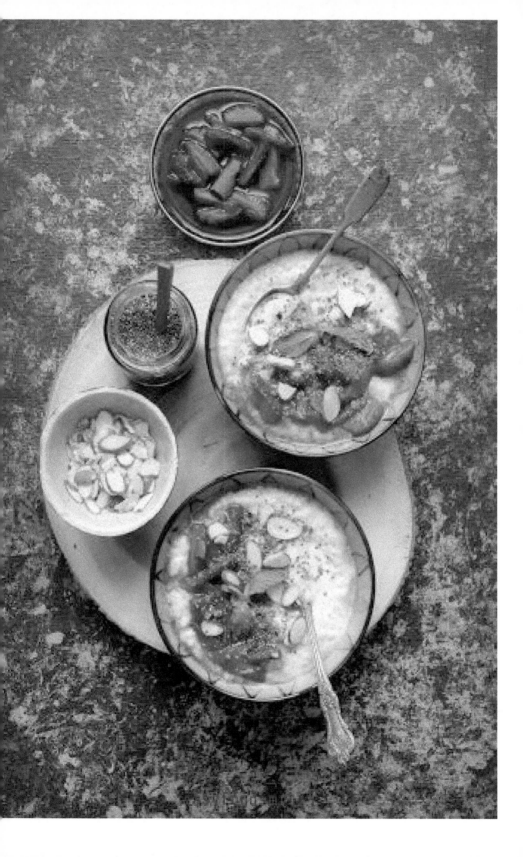

Bread Pudding with Raisins

Ready in about: 1 hour

Servings: 8

Per serving: Calories: 474; Fat: 12.2g; Carbs: 72g; Protein: 14.4g

Ingredients

- 8 cups day-old bread, cubed
- 1 cup brown sugar
- 8 cups coconut milk
- 1 teaspoon vanilla extract
- 2 teaspoons ground cinnamon
- 4 tablespoons rum
- 1 cup raisins

Directions

1. Start by preheating your oven to 360 degrees F. Lightly oil a casserole dish with a nonstick cooking spray.
2. Place the cubed bread in the prepared casserole dish.
3. In a mixing bowl, thoroughly combine the sugar, milk, vanilla, cinnamon, rum, and raisins. Pour the custard evenly over the bread cubes.
4. Let it soak for about 15 minutes.
5. Bake in the preheated oven for about 45 minutes or until the top is golden and set
6. Bon appétit!

Rye Porridge with Blueberry Topping

Ready in about: 15 minutes

Servings: 6

Per serving: Calories: 359; Fat: 11g; Carbs: 56.1g; Protein: 12.1g

Ingredients

- 2 cups rye flakes
- 2 cups water
- 2 cups coconut milk
- 2 cups fresh blueberries
- 2 tablespoons coconut oil
- 12 dates, pitted

Directions

1. Add the rye flakes, water and coconut milk to a deep saucepan; bring to a boil over medium-high. Turn the heat to a simmer and let it cook for 5 to 6 minutes.
2. In a blender or food processor, puree the blueberries with coconut oil and dates.
3. Ladle into three bowls and garnish with the blueberry topping.
4. Bon appétit!

Easy Spinach Ricotta Pasta

Ready in about: 05 minutes

Servings: 4

Per serving: Calories277, Total Fat 18. 9g, Saturated Fat 15. 2g, Cholesterol 16mg, Sodium 191mg, Total Carbohydrate 23. 8g, Dietary Fiber 1. 2g, Total Sugars 1. 4g, Protein 5. 1g

Ingredients:

- ½ cup pasta
- 1 cup vegetable broth
- 1/2 lb. uncooked tagliatelle
- 1 tablespoon coconut oil
- ½ teaspoon garlic powder
- ¼ cup almond milk
- ½ cup whole milk ricotta
- 1/8 teaspoon salt
- Freshly cracked pepper
- ¼ cup chopped spinach

Directions:

1. Add the vegetable broth, tagliatelle, spinach, salt, some freshly cracked pepper, and the pasta. Place lid on Instant Pot and lock into place to seal. Pressure Cook on High Pressure for 4 minutes. Use Quick Pressure Release.

2. Prepare the ricotta sauce. Mince the garlic and add it to a large skillet with coconut oil. Cook over Medium-Low heat for 1-2 minutes, or just until soft and fragrant (but not browned). Add the almond milk and ricotta, then stir until relatively smooth (the ricotta may be slightly grainy). Allow the sauce to heat through and come to a low simmer. The sauce will thicken slightly as it simmers. Once it's thick enough to coat the spoon (3-5 minutes), season with salt and pepper.

3. Add the cooked and drained pasta to the sauce and toss to coat. If the sauce becomes too thick or dry, add a small amount of the reserved pasta cooking water. Serve warm.

Pasta with Peppers

Preparation Time: 5 minutes

Servings: 4

Per serving: Calories 291, Total Fat 6. 2g, Saturated Fat 2. 9g, Cholesterol 61mg, Sodium 994mg, Total Carbohydrate 43. 7g, Dietary Fiber 1g, Total Sugars 3. 5g, Protein 15. 1g

Ingredients:
- 3 cups spaghetti sauce
- 2 cups vegetable broth
- 1 tablespoon dried Italian seasoning blend
- 2 cups bell pepper strips
- 2 cups dried pasta
- 2 cups shredded Romano cheese

Directions:
1. Press the button Sauté. Set it for High, and set the time for 10 minutes.
2. Mix the sauce, broth, and seasoning blend in an Instant Pot. Cook, turn off the Sauté function; stir in the bell pepper strips and pasta. Lock the lid onto the pot.
3. Press Pressure Cook on Max Pressure for 5 minutes with the Keep Warm setting off.
4. Use the Quick Release method to bring the pot pressure back to normal. Unlatch the lid and open

the cooker. Stir in the shredded Romano cheese. Set the lid askew over the pot and set aside for 5 minutes to melt the cheese and let the pasta continue to absorb excess liquid. Serve by the big spoon.

5. Bon Appetit!!

Creamy Penne with Vegetables

Ready in about: 05 minutes

Servings: 2

Per serving: Calories 381, Total Fat 13. 2g, Saturated Fat 8. 7g, Cholesterol 56mg, Sodium 1006mg, Total Carbohydrate 52. 3g, Dietary Fiber 4. 7g, Total Sugars 8. 6g, Protein 15. 3g

Ingredients:
- ½ tablespoon butter
- 1 cup penne
- 1 small onion
- ½ teaspoon garlic powder
- 1 carrot
- ½ red bell pepper
- ½ pumpkin
- 2 cups vegetable broth
- 2 oz. coconut cream
- 1/8 cup grated Parmesan cheese
- 1/8 teaspoon salt and pepper to taste
- Dash hot sauce, optional
- ¼ cup cauliflower florets

Directions:
1. Set Instant Pot to Sauté. Add the butter and allow it to melt. Add the onion and garlic powder and cook for 2 minutes. Stir regularly. Add the carrot,

red pepper and pumpkin, and cauliflower to the pot.

2. Add penne, vegetable broth, coconut cream, salt, and pepper, then add hot sauce.

3. Lock the lid and make sure the vent is closed. Set Instant Pot to Manual or Pressure Cook on High Pressure for 10 minutes. When cooking time ends, release pressure and wait for steam to completely stop before opening the lid.

4. Stir in cheese, sprinkle a bit on top of the pasta when you serve it.

Baked Cheesy Spaghetti Squash

Ready in about: 40 minutes

Servings: 8

Ingredients

- 4 lbs spaghetti squash
- 2 tbsps coconut oil
- Salt and black pepper to taste
- 4 tbsps melted plant butter
- 1 tbsp garlic powder
- 2/5 tsp chili powder
- 2 cups coconut cream
- 4 oz cashew cream cheese
- 2 cups plant-based mozzarella
- 4 oz grated plant-based Parmesan
- 4 tbsps fresh cilantro, chopped
- Olive oil for drizzling

Directions

1. Preheat oven to 350 F.

2. Cut the squash in halves lengthwise and spoon out the seeds and fiber. Place on a baking dish, brush with coconut oil, and season with salt and pepper. Bake for 30 minutes. Remove and use two forks to shred the flesh into strands.

3. Empty the spaghetti strands into a bowl and mix with plant butter, garlic and chili powders, coconut cream, cream cheese, half of the plant-based mozzarella, and plant-based Parmesan cheeses. Spoon the mixture into the squash cups and sprinkle with the remaining mozzarella cheese. Bake further for 5 minutes. Sprinkle with cilantro and drizzle with some oil. Serve.

Vegan Mushroom Pizza

Ready in about: 35 minutes

Servings: 8

Ingredients

- 4 tsps plant butter
- 2 cups chopped button mushrooms
- 1 cup sliced mixed bell peppers
- Salt and black pepper to taste
- 2 pizza crust
- 2 cups tomato sauce
- 2 cups plant-based Parmesan cheese
- 10 basil leaves

Directions

1. Melt plant butter in a skillet and sauté mushrooms and bell peppers for 10 minutes until softened. Season with salt and black pepper. Put the pizza crust on a pizza pan, spread the tomato sauce all over, and scatter vegetables evenly on top. Sprinkle with plant-based Parmesan cheese. Bake for 20 minutes until the cheese has melted. Garnish with basil and serve.

2. Enjoy!

Eggplant Fries with Chili Aioli & Beet Salad

Ready in about: 35 minutes

Servings: 8

Ingredients

Eggplant Fries:

- 4 tbsps flax seed powder

- 4 eggplants, sliced
- 4 cups almond flour
- Salt and black pepper to taste
- 4 tbsps olive oil

Beet salad:

- 7 oz beets, peeled and thinly cut

- 7 oz red cabbage, grated
- 4 tbsps fresh cilantro
- 4 tbsps olive oil
- 2 tbsps freshly squeezed lime juice
- Salt and black pepper to taste

Spicy Aioli:

- 2 tbsps flax seed powder

- 4 garlic cloves, minced

- 5 cups light olive oil
- 1 tsp red chili flakes
- 2 tbsps freshly squeezed lemon juice
- 6 tbsps dairy-free yogurt

Directions

1. Preheat oven to 400 F. In a bowl, combine the flax seed powder with 6 tbsps water and allow sitting to thicken for 5 minutes. In a deep plate, mix almond flour, salt, and black pepper. Dip the eggplant slices into the vegan "flax egg," then in the almond flour, and then in the vegan "flax egg," and finally in the flour mixture. Place the eggplants on a greased baking sheet and drizzle with olive oil. Bake until the fries are crispy and brown, about 15 minutes.

2. For the aioli, mix the flax seed powder with 3 tbsps water in a bowl and set aside to thicken for 5 minutes. Whisk in garlic while pouring in the olive oil gradually. Stir in red chili flakes, salt, black pepper, lemon juice, and dairy-free yogurt. Adjust the taste with salt, garlic, or yogurt as desired.

3. For the beet salad, in a salad bowl, combine the beets, red cabbage, cilantro, olive oil, lime juice, salt, and black pepper. Use two spoons to toss the ingredients until properly combined. Serve the eggplant fries with the chili aioli and beet salad.

Mushroom Lettuce Wraps

Ready in about: 25 minutes

Servings: 8

Ingredients

- 4 tbsps plant butter
- 8 oz baby Bella mushrooms, sliced
- 3 lbs tofu, crumbled
- 2 iceberg lettuce, leaves extracted
- 2 cups grated plant-based cheddar
- 2 large tomatoes, sliced

Directions

1. Melt the plant butter in a skillet, add in mushrooms and sauté until browned and tender, about 6 minutes. Transfer to a plate. Add the tofu to the skillet and cook until brown, about 10 minutes. Spoon the tofu and mushrooms into the lettuce leaves, sprinkle with the plant-based cheddar cheese, and share the tomato slices on top. Serve the burger immediately.

DINNER

White Bean and Cabbage Stew

Ready in about: 5 minutes

Servings: 8

Per serving: Calories: 150 Cal Fat: 0.7 g Carbs: 27 g Protein: 7 g Fiber: 9.4 g

Ingredients:

- 6 cups cooked great northern beans
- pounds potatoes, peeled, cut into large dice
- 2 large white onions, peeled, chopped
- 1 head of cabbage, chopped
- 6 ribs celery, chopped
- 8 medium carrots, peeled, sliced
- 14.5 ounces diced tomatoes
- 2/3 cup pearled barley
- 2 teaspoons minced garlic
- 1 teaspoon ground black pepper
- 2 bay leaves
- 2 teaspoons dried thyme
- 1 teaspoon crushed rosemary
- 2 teaspoons salt
- 1 teaspoon caraway seeds
- 2 tablespoons chopped parsley
- 16 cups vegetable broth

Directions:

1. Switch on the slow cooker, then add all the ingredients except for salt, parsley, tomatoes, and beans and stir until mixed.
2. Shut the slow cooker with a lid, and cook for 7 hours at a low heat setting until cooked.
3. Then stir in remaining ingredients, stir until combined, and continue cooking for 1 hour.
4. Serve straight away

Cabbage Stew

Ready in about: 60 minutes

Servings: 12

Per serving: Calories: 182 Cal Fat: 8.3 g Carbs: 27 g Protein: 5.5 g Fiber: 9.4 g

Ingredients:
- 24 ounces cooked Cannellini beans
- 16 ounces smoked tofu, firm, sliced
- 2 medium cabbage, chopped
- 2 large white onions, peeled, julienned
- 5 teaspoons minced garlic
- 2 tablespoons sweet paprika
- 10 tablespoons tomato paste
- 6 teaspoons smoked paprika
- 2/3 teaspoon ground black pepper
- 4 teaspoons dried thyme
- 1/3 teaspoon salt
- 1 tsp ground coriander
- 6 bay leaves
- 8 tablespoons olive oil
- 2 cups vegetable broth

Directions:
1. Take a large saucepan, place it over medium heat, add 3 tablespoons oil and when hot, add onion and garlic and cook for 3 minutes or until sauté.

2. Add cabbage, pour in water, simmer for 10 minutes or until softened, then stir in all the spices and continue cooking for 30 minutes.
3. Add beans and tomato paste, pour in water, stir until mixed and cook for 15 minutes until thoroughly cooked.
4. Take a separate skillet pan, add 1 tablespoon oil and when hot, add tofu slices and cook for 5 minutes until golden brown on both sides.
5. Serve cooked cabbage stew with fried tofu.

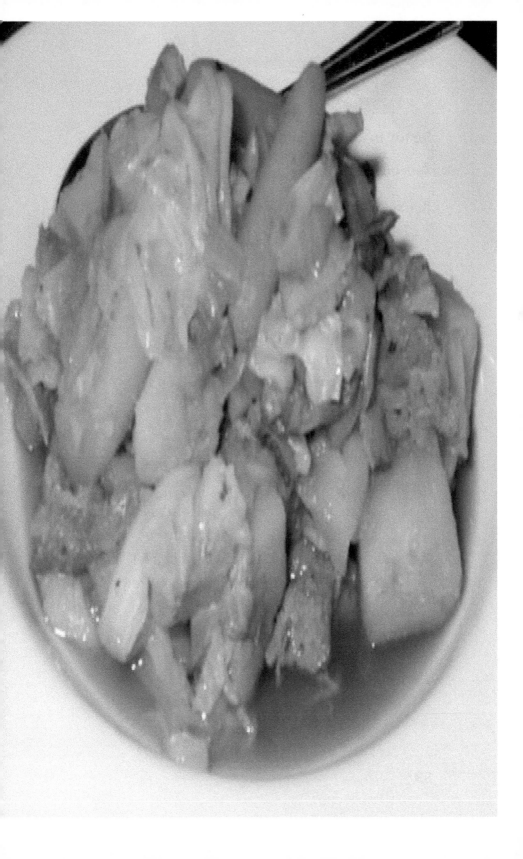

Eggplant, Onion, and Tomato Stew

Ready in about: 5 minutes

Servings: 4

Per serving: Calories: 88 Cal Fat: 1 g Carbs: 21 g Protein: 3 g Fiber: 6 g

Ingredients:
- 7 cups cubed eggplant
- 2 cups diced white onion
- 4 cups diced tomatoes
- 2 teaspoons ground cumin
- 1/4 teaspoon ground cayenne pepper
- 2 teaspoons salt
- 2 cups tomato sauce
- 1 cup water

Directions:
1. Switch on the instant pot, place all the ingredients in it, stir until mixed, and seal the pot.
2. Press the 'manual' button and cook for 5 minutes at a high-pressure setting until cooked.
3. When done, do quick pressure release, open the instant pot, and stir the stew.
4. Serve straight away.
5. Enjoy!

Portobello Mushroom Stew

Ready in about: 10 minutes

Servings: 8

Per serving: Calories: 447 Cal Fat: 36 g Carbs: 24 g Protein: 11 g Fiber: 2 g

Ingredients:
- 16 cups vegetable broth
- 2 cups dried wild mushrooms
- 2 cups dried chickpeas
- 6 cups chopped potato
- 4 cups chopped carrots
- 2 cups corn kernels
- 4 cups diced white onions
- 2 tablespoons minced parsley
- 6 cups chopped zucchini
- 2 tablespoons minced rosemary
- 3 teaspoons ground black pepper
- 2 teaspoons dried sage
- 4/3 teaspoons salt
- 2 teaspoons dried oregano
- 6 tablespoons soy sauce
- 3 teaspoons liquid smoke
- 16 ounces tomato paste

Directions:

1. Switch on the slow cooker, add all the ingredients to it, and stir until mixed.
2. Shut the cooker with a lid and cook for 10 hours at a high heat setting until cooked.
3. Serve straight away.

Oregano Chickpeas

Ready in about: 10 minutes

Servings: 12

Ingredients

- 2 tsps olive oil
- 2 onions, cut into half-moon slices
- 4 (14.5-oz) cans chickpeas
- 1 cup vegetable broth
- 4 tsps dried oregano
- Salt and black pepper to taste

Directions

1. Heat the oil in a skillet over medium heat. Cook the onion for 3 minutes. Stir in chickpeas, broth, oregano, salt, and pepper. Bring to a boil, then lower the heat and simmer for 10 minutes. Serve.

Matcha-Infused Tofu Rice

Ready in about: 35 minutes

Servings: 8

Ingredients

- 8 matcha tea bags
- 3 cups brown rice
- 4 tbsps canola oil
- 16 oz extra-firm tofu, chopped
- 6 green onions, minced
- 4 cups snow peas, cut diagonally
- 2 tbsps fresh lemon juice
- 2 tsps grated lemon zest
- Salt and black pepper to taste

Directions

1. Boil 3 cups of water in a pot. Place in the tea bags and turn the heat off. Let sit for 7 minutes. Discard the bags. Wash the rice and put it into the tea. Cook for 20 minutes over medium heat. Drain and set aside.

2. Heat the oil in a skillet over medium heat. Fry the tofu for 5 minutes until golden. Stir in green onions and snow peas and cook for another 3 minutes. Mix in lemon juice and lemon zest. Place

the rice in a serving bowl and mix it in the tofu mixture. Adjust the seasoning with salt and pepper. Serve right away.

Savory Seitan & Bell Pepper Rice

Ready in about: 35 minutes

Servings: 4

Ingredients

- 4 cups water
- 2 cups long-grain brown rice
- 4 tbsps olive oil
- 2 onions, chopped
- 4 garlic cloves, minced
- 16 oz seitan, chopped
- 2 green bell peppers, chopped
- 2 tsps dried basil
- 1 tsp ground fennel seeds
- ½ tsp crushed red pepper
- Salt and black pepper to taste

Directions

1. Bring water to a boil in a pot. Place in rice and lower the heat. Simmer for 20 minutes.

2. Heat the oil in a skillet over medium heat. Sauté the onion for 3 minutes until translucent. Add in the seitan and bell pepper and cook for another 5 minutes. Stir in basil, fennel, red pepper, salt, and black pepper. Once the rice is ready, remove it to a bowl. Add in seitan mixture and toss to combine. Serve.

Green Pea & Lemon Couscous

Ready in about: 15 minutes

Servings: 12

Ingredients

- 2 cups green peas
- 4 cups vegetable stock
- Juice and zest of 1 lemon
- 4 tbsps chopped fresh thyme
- 3 cups couscous
- ½ cup chopped fresh parsley

Directions

1. Pour the vegetable stock, lemon juice, thyme, salt, and pepper into a pot. Bring to a boil, then add in green peas and couscous. Turn the heat off and let sit covered for 5 minutes until the liquid has absorbed. Fluff the couscous using a fork and mix in the lemon and parsley. Serve immediately.

Acorn Squash, Chickpea, and Couscous Soup

Ready in about: 20 minutes

Servings: 8

Per serving: Calories: 378; Fat: 11g; Carbs: 60.1g; Protein: 10.9g

Ingredients
- 4 tablespoons olive oil
- 2 shallots, chopped
- 2 carrots, trimmed and chopped
- 4 cups acorn squash, chopped
- 2 stalk celery, chopped
- 2 teaspoons garlic, finely chopped
- 2 teaspoons dried rosemary, chopped
- 2 teaspoons dried thyme, chopped
- 4 cups cream of onion soup
- 4 cups water
- 2 cups dry couscous
- Sea salt and ground black pepper, to taste
- 1 teaspoon red pepper flakes
- 12 ounces canned chickpeas, drained
- 4 tablespoons fresh lemon juice

Directions

1. In a heavy-bottomed pot, heat the olive over medium-high heat. Now, sauté the shallot, carrot, acorn squash, and celery for about 3 minutes or until the vegetables are just tender.

2. Add in the garlic, rosemary, and thyme, and continue to sauté for 1 minute or until aromatic.

3. Then, stir in the soup, water, couscous, salt, black pepper, and red pepper flakes; bring to a boil. Immediately reduce the heat to a simmer and let it cook for 12 minutes.

4. Fold in the canned chickpeas; continue to simmer until heated through or about 5 minutes more.

5. Ladle into individual bowls and drizzle with the lemon juice over the top. Bon appétit!

Cabbage Soup with Garlic Crostini

Ready in about: 1 hour

Servings: 8

Per serving: Calories: 408; Fat: 23.1g; Carbs: 37.6g; Protein: 11.8g

Ingredients

Soup:

- 4 tablespoons olive oil
- 2 medium leek, chopped
- 2 cups turnip, chopped
- 2 parsnips, chopped
- 2 carrots, chopped
- 4 cups cabbage, shredded
- 4 garlic cloves, finely chopped
- 8 cups vegetable broth
- 4 bay leaves
- Sea salt and ground black pepper, to taste
- 1/2 teaspoon cumin seeds
- 1 teaspoon mustard seeds
- 2 teaspoons dried basil
- 4 tomatoes, pureed
- Crostini:
- 16 slices of baguette
- 4 heads garlic
- 8 tablespoons extra-virgin olive oil

Directions

1. In a soup pot, heat 2 tablespoons of the olive over medium-high heat. Now, sauté the leek, turnip, parsnip, and carrot for about 4 minutes or until the vegetables are crisp-tender.
2. Add in the garlic and cabbage and continue to sauté for 1 minute or until aromatic.
3. Then, stir in the vegetable broth, bay leaves, salt, black pepper, cumin seeds, mustard seeds, dried basil, and pureed tomatoes; bring to a boil. Immediately reduce the heat to a simmer and let it cook for about 20 minutes.
4. Meanwhile, preheat your oven to 375 degrees F. Now, roast the garlic and baguette slices for about 15 minutes. Remove the crostini from the oven.
5. Continue baking the garlic for 45 minutes more or until very tender. Allow the garlic to cool.
6. Now, cut each head of the garlic using a sharp serrated knife in order to separate all the cloves.
7. Squeeze the roasted garlic cloves out of their skins. Mash the garlic pulp with 4 tablespoons of the extra-virgin olive oil.
8. Spread the roasted garlic mixture evenly on the tops of the crostini. Serve with warm soup. Bon appétit!

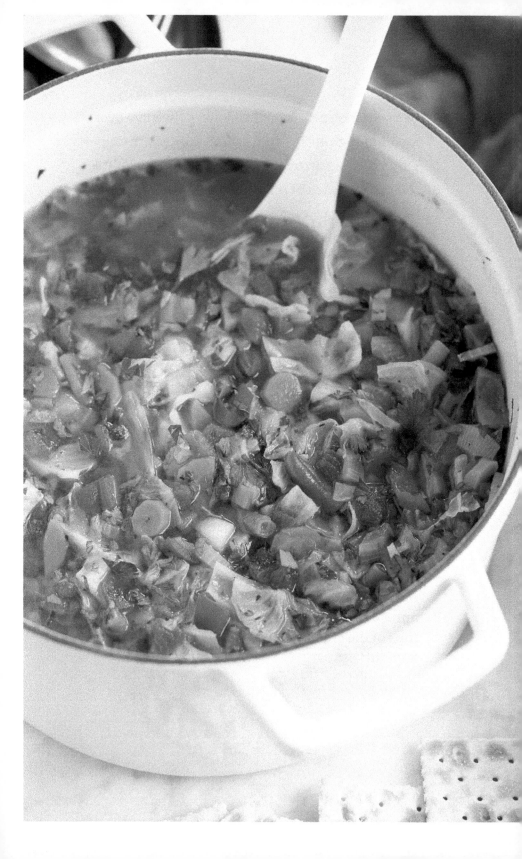

Classic Cream of Broccoli Soup

Ready in about: 35 minutes

Servings: 8

Per serving: Calories: 334; Fat: 24.5g; Carbs: 22.5g; Protein: 10.2g

Ingredients

- 4 tablespoons olive oil
- 2 pounds broccoli florets
- 2 onions, chopped
- 2 celeries rib, chopped
- 2 parsnips, chopped
- 2 teaspoons garlic, chopped
- 6 cups vegetable broth
- 1 teaspoon dried dill
- 1 teaspoon dried oregano
- Sea salt and ground black pepper, to taste
- 4 tablespoons flaxseed meal
- 2 cups full-fat coconut milk

Directions

1. In a heavy-bottomed pot, heat the olive oil over medium-high heat. Now, sauté the broccoli onion, celery, and parsnip for about 5 minutes, stirring periodically.
2. Add in the garlic and continue sautéing for 1 minute or until fragrant.

3. Then, stir in the vegetable broth, dill, oregano, salt, and black pepper; bring to a boil. Immediately reduce the heat to a simmer and let it cook for about 20 minutes.
4. Puree the soup using an immersion blender until creamy and uniform.
5. Return the pureed mixture to the pot. Fold in the flaxseed meal and coconut milk; continue to simmer until heated through or about 5 minutes.
6. Ladle into four serving bowls and enjoy!

Traditional French Onion Soup

Ready in about: 1 hour 30 minutes

Servings: 8

Per serving: Calories: 129; Fat: 8.6g; Carbs: 7.4g; Protein: 6.3g

Ingredients

- 4 tablespoons olive oil
- 4 large yellow onions, thinly sliced
- 4 thyme sprigs, chopped
- 4 rosemary sprigs, chopped
- 4 teaspoons balsamic vinegar
- 8 cups vegetable stock
- Sea salt and ground black pepper, to taste

Directions

1. In a or Dutch oven, heat the olive oil over moderate heat. Now, cook the onions with thyme, rosemary, and 1 teaspoon of sea salt for about 2 minutes.
2. Now, turn the heat to medium-low and continue cooking until the onions caramelize or about 50 minutes.
3. Add in the balsamic vinegar and continue to cook for a further 15 more. Add in the stock, salt, and black pepper, and continue simmering for 20 to 25 minutes.
4. Serve with toasted bread and enjoy!

DESSERTS

Salted Caramel Chocolate Cups

Preparation Time: 5 minutes

Servings: 12

Per Serving: Calories: 80 Cal Fat: 5 g Carbs: 10 g Protein: 1 g Fiber: 0.5 g

Ingredients:
- ½ teaspoon sea salt granules
- 2 cups dark chocolate chips, unsweetened
- 4 teaspoons coconut oil
- 12 tablespoons caramel sauce

Directions:
1. Take a heatproof bowl, add chocolate chips and oil, stir until mixed, then microwave for 1 minute until melted, stir chocolate and continue heating in the microwave for 30 seconds.
2. Take twelve mini muffin tins, line them with muffin liners, spoon a little bit of chocolate mixture into the tins, spread the chocolate in the bottom and along the sides, and freeze for 10 minutes until set.
3. Then fill each cup with ½ tablespoon of caramel sauce, cover with remaining chocolate and freeze for another 2salt0 minutes until set.
4. When ready to eat, peel off liner from the cup, sprinkle with sauce, and serve.

Chocolate & Almond Butter Barks

Ready in about: 15-30 minutes

Servings: 8

Per serving: Calories 279 Fats 28. 1g Carbs 8. 6g Protein 4. 4g

Ingredients:

- 2/3 cup coconut oil, melted
- ½ cup almond butter, melted
- 4 tbsps unsweetened coconut flakes.
- 2 tsps pure maple syrup
- A pinch of ground rock salt
- ½ cup unsweetened cocoa nibs

Directions:

1. Line a baking tray with baking paper and set it aside.
2. In a medium bowl, mix the coconut oil, almond butter, coconut flakes, maple syrup, and then fold in the rock salt and cocoa nibs.
3. Pour and spread the mixture on the baking sheet, chill in the refrigerator for 20 minutes or until firm.
4. Remove the dessert, break it into shards, and enjoy it immediately.
5. Preserve extras in the refrigerator.

Mini Berry Tarts

Ready in about: 15-30 minutes
Servings: 4
Per serving: Calories 545 Fats 33. 5g Carbs 53. 6g Protein 10. 6g

Ingredients:

For the pie crust:

- 4 tbsps flax seed powder + 12 tbsps water
- 1/3 cup whole-wheat flour + more for dusting
- ½ tsp salt
- ¼ cup plant butter, cold and crumbled
- 3 tbsps pure malt syrup
- 1 ½ tsps vanilla extract
- For the filling:
- 6 oz cashew cream
- 6 tbsps pure date sugar
- ¾ tsp vanilla extract
- 1 cup mixed frozen berries

Directions:

1. Preheat the oven to 350 F and grease a mini pie pan with cooking spray.
2. In a medium bowl, mix the flax seed powder with water and allow soaking for 5 minutes.
3. In a large bowl, combine the flour and salt. Add the butter, and using an electric hand mixer,

whisk until crumbly. Pour in the flax egg, malt syrup, vanilla, and mix until smooth dough forms.

4. Flatten the dough on a flat surface, cover with plastic wrap, and refrigerate for 1 hour.

5. After, lightly dust a working surface with some flour, remove the dough onto the surface, and using a rolling pin, flatten the dough into a 1-inch diameter circle,

6. Use a large cookie cutter, cut out rounds of the dough and fit into the pie pans. Use a knife to trim the edges of the pan. Lay a parchment paper on the dough cups, pour on some baking beans, and bake in the oven until golden brown, 15 to 20 minutes.

7. Remove the pans from the oven, pour out the baking beans, and allow cooling.

8. In a medium bowl, mix the cashew cream, date sugar, and vanilla extract.

9. Divide the mixture into the tart cups and top with berries. Serve immediately.

Cardamom Coconut Fat Bombs

Preparation Time: 5minutes

Servings: 12

Per serving: Calories: 687, Total Fat: 54.5g, Saturated Fat: 27.4 g, Total Carbs: 9g, Dietary Fiber: 2g, Sugar: 4g, Protein: 38g, Sodium: 883 mg

Ingredients:
- 1 cup unsweetened grated coconut
- 6 oz. unsalted butter, room temperature
- 1/2 tsp green cardamom powder
- 1 tsp vanilla extract
- ½ tsp cinnamon powder

Directions:
1. Pour the grated coconut into a skillet and roast until lightly brown. Set aside to cool.
2. In a bowl, combine the butter, half of the coconut, cardamom, vanilla, and cinnamon.
3. Use your hands to form bite-size balls from the mixture and roll each in the remaining coconut.
4. Refrigerate the balls until ready to serve.

Vanilla Brownies

Ready in about: 30 minutes + chilling time

Servings: 8

Ingredients

- 4 tbsps flaxseed powder
- 1/2 cup cocoa powder
- 1 cup almond flour
- 1 tsp baking powder
- 1 cup erythritol
- 20 tablespoons plant butter
- 4 oz dairy-free dark chocolate
- 1 teaspoon vanilla extract

Directions

1. Preheat oven to 375 F and line a baking sheet with parchment paper. Mix the flaxseed powder with 6 tbsps water in a bowl and allow thickening for 5 minutes. In a separate bowl, mix cocoa powder, almond flour, baking powder, and erythritol until no lumps. In another bowl, add the plant butter and dark chocolate and melt both in the microwave for 30 seconds to 1 minute.

2. Whisk the vegan "flax egg" and vanilla into the chocolate mixture, then pour the mixture into the

dry ingredients. Combine evenly. Pour the batter onto the paper-lined baking sheet and bake for 20 minutes. Cool completely and refrigerate for 2 hours. When ready, slice into squares and serve.

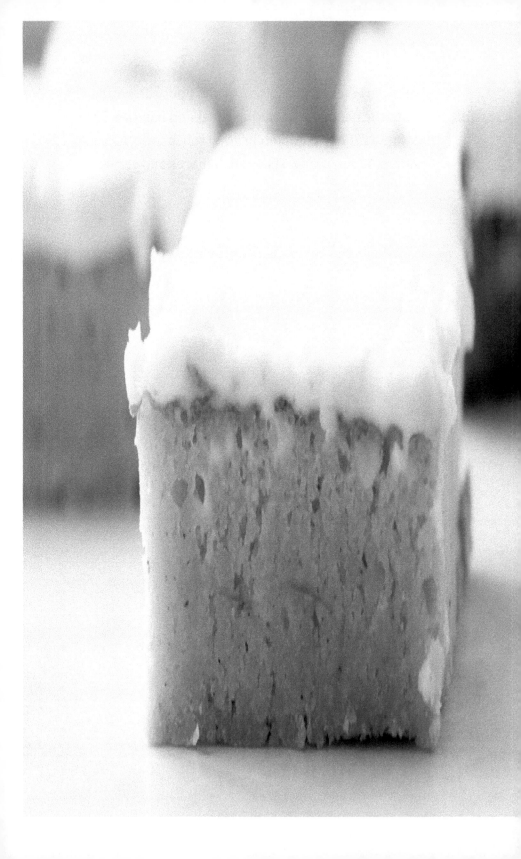

Lime Avocado Ice Cream

Ready in about: 10 minutes

Servings: 8

Ingredients

- 4 large avocados, pitted
- Juice and zest of 3 limes
- 2/3 cup erythritol
- 4 cups coconut cream
- ½ tsp vanilla extract

Directions

1. In a blender, combine the avocado pulp, lime juice and zest, erythritol, coconut cream, and vanilla extract. Process until the mixture is smooth. Pour the mixture into your ice cream maker and freeze based on the manufacturer's instructions. When ready, remove and scoop the ice cream into bowls. Serve immediately.

2. Enjoy

Vanilla White Chocolate Pudding

Ready in about: 20 minutes+ cooling time

Servings: 8

Ingredients

- 6 tbsps flaxseed + 9 tbsps water
- 6 tbsps cornstarch
- 2 cups cashew cream
- 5 cups almond milk
- 1 pure date sugar
- 2 tbsps vanilla caviar
- 12 oz white chocolate chips
- Whipped coconut cream
- Sliced bananas and raspberries

Directions

1. In a small bowl, mix the flaxseed powder with water and allow thickening for 5 minutes to make the vegan "flax egg." In a large bowl, whisk the cornstarch and cashew cream until smooth. Beat in the vegan "flax egg" until well combined.

2. Pour the almond milk into a pot and whisk in the date sugar. Cook over medium heat while frequently stirring until the sugar dissolves.

Reduce the heat to low and simmer until steamy and bubbly around the edges.

3. Pour half of the almond milk mixture into the vegan "flax egg" mix, whisk well and pour this mixture into the remaining milk content in the pot. Whisk continuously until well combined. Bring the new mixture to a boil over medium heat while still frequently stirring and scraping all the pot's corners, 2 minutes.

4. Turn the heat off, stir in the vanilla caviar, then the white chocolate chips until melted. Spoon the mixture into a bowl, allow cooling for 2 minutes, cover with plastic wraps, making sure to press the plastic onto the surface of the pudding, and refrigerate for 4 hours. Remove the pudding from the fridge, take off the plastic wrap, and whip for about a minute. Spoon the dessert into serving cups, swirl some coconut whipping cream on top, and top with the bananas and raspberries. Enjoy.

Southern Apple Cobbler with Raspberries

Ready in about: 50 minutes

Servings: 8

Ingredients

- 6 apples, chopped
- 4 tbsps pure date sugar
- 2 cups fresh raspberries
- 4 tbsps unsalted plant butter
- 1 cup whole-wheat flour
- 2 cups toasted rolled oats
- 4 tbsps pure date sugar
- 2 tsps cinnamon powder

Directions

1. Preheat the oven to 350 F and grease a baking dish with some plant butter.

2. Add apples, date sugar, and 3 tbsps of water to a pot. Cook over low heat until the date sugar melts and then mix in the raspberries. Cook until the fruits soften, 10 minutes. Pour and spread the fruit mixture into the baking dish and set aside.

3. In a blender, add the plant butter, flour, oats, date sugar, and cinnamon powder. Pulse a few times until crumbly. Spoon and spread the mixture on

the fruit mix until evenly layered. Bake in the oven for 25 to 30 minutes or until golden brown on top. Remove the dessert, allow cooling for 2 minutes, and serve.

Mushroom and Cannellini Bean "Meatballs"

Ready in about: 15 minutes

Servings: 8

Per serving: Calories: 195; Fat: 14.1g; Carbs: 13.2g; Protein: 3.9g

Ingredients

- 8 tablespoons olive oil
- 2 cups button mushrooms, chopped
- 2 shallot, chopped
- 4 garlic cloves, crushed
- 2 cups canned or boiled cannellini beans, drained
- 2 cups quinoa, cooked
- Sea salt and ground black pepper, to taste
- 2 teaspoons smoked paprika
- 1 teaspoon red pepper flakes
- 2 teaspoons mustard seeds
- 1 teaspoon dried dill

Directions

1. Heat 2 tablespoons of the olive oil in a nonstick skillet. Once hot, cook the mushrooms and shallot for 3 minutes or until just tender.
2. Add in the garlic, beans, quinoa and spices. Mix to combine well and then, shape the mixture into equal balls using oiled hands.

3. Then, heat the remaining 2 tablespoons of the olive oil in a nonstick skillet over medium heat. Once hot, fry the meatballs for about 10 minutes until golden brown on all sides.

4. Serve with cocktail sticks.

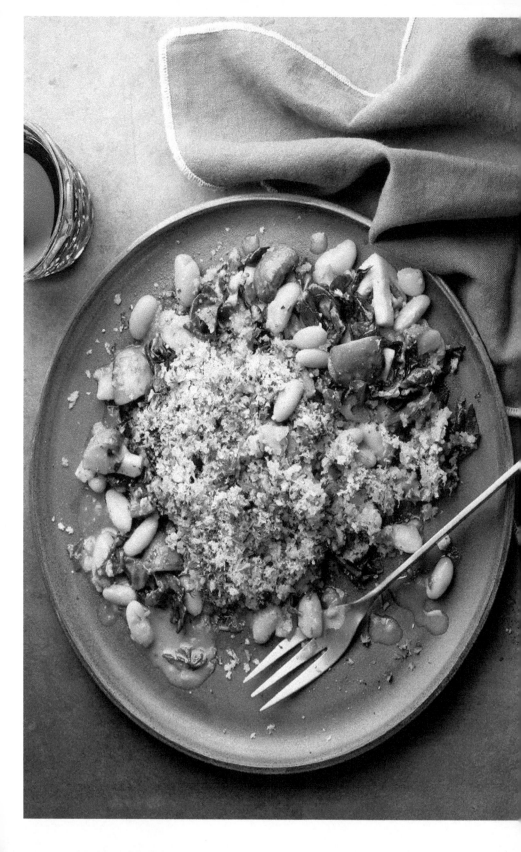

Stuffed Jalapeño Bites

Ready in about: 15 minutes

Servings: 12

Per serving: Calories: 108; Fat: 6.6g; Carbs: 7.3g; Protein: 5.3g

Ingredients

- 1 cup raw sunflower seeds, soaked overnight, and drained
- 8 tablespoons scallions, chopped
- 2 teaspoons garlic, minced
- 6 tablespoons nutritional yeast
- 1 cup cream of onion soup
- 1 teaspoon cayenne pepper
- 1 teaspoon mustard seeds
- 24 jalapeños, halved and seeded
- 1 cup breadcrumbs

Directions

1. In your food processor or high-speed blender, blitz raw sunflower seeds, scallions, garlic, nutritional yeast, soup, cayenne pepper, and mustard seeds until well combined.
2. Spoon the mixture into the jalapeños and top them with the breadcrumbs.

3. Bake in the preheated oven at 400 degrees F for about 13 minutes or until the peppers have softened. Serve warm.
4. Bon appétit!

Roasted Root Vegetables

Ready in about: 35 minutes

Servings: 12

Per serving: Calories: 261; Fat: 18.2g; Carbs: 23.3g; Protein: 2.3g

Ingredients

- 1/2 cup olive oil
- 4 carrots, peeled and cut into 3-inch pieces
- 4 parsnips, peeled and cut into 3-inch pieces
- 2 celeries stalk, peeled, and cut into 3-inch pieces
- 2 pound sweet potatoes, peeled and cut into 3-inch pieces
- 1/2 cup olive oil
- 2 teaspoons mustard seeds
- 1 teaspoon basil
- 1 teaspoon oregano
- 2 teaspoons red pepper flakes
- 2 teaspoons dried thyme
- Sea salt and ground black pepper, to taste

Directions

1. Toss the vegetables with the remaining ingredients until well coated.
2. Roast the vegetables in the preheated oven at 400 degrees F for about 35 minutes, stirring halfway through the cooking time.
3. Taste, adjust the seasonings, and serve warm.
4. Bon appétit!

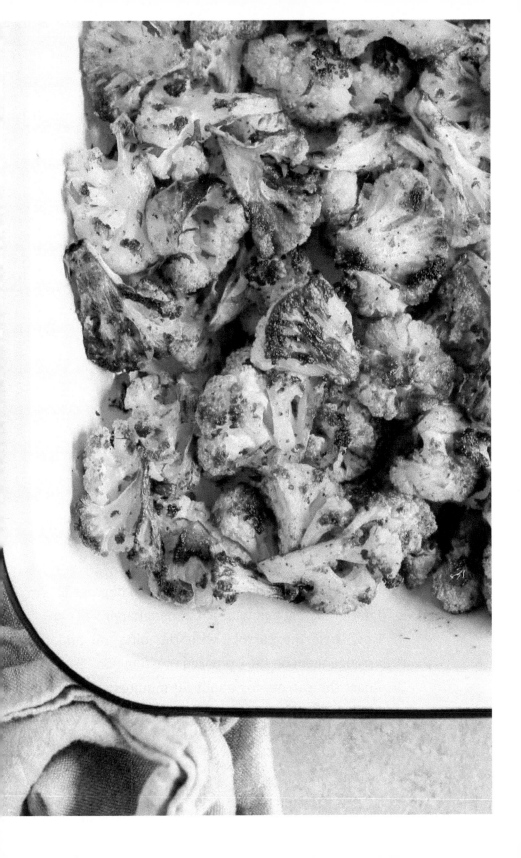

Roasted Carrot and Bean Dip

Ready in about: 55 minutes

Servings: 20

Per serving: Calories: 121; Fat: 8.3g; Carbs: 11.2g; Protein: 2.8g

Ingredients

- 3 pounds carrots, trimmed
- 4 tablespoons olive oil
- 8 tablespoons tahini
- 16 ounces canned cannellini beans, drained
- 2 teaspoons garlic, chopped
- 4 tablespoons lemon juice
- 4 tablespoons soy sauce
- Sea salt and ground black pepper, to taste
- 1 teaspoon paprika
- 1 teaspoon dried dill
- 1/2 cup pepitas, toasted

Directions

1. Begin by preheating your oven to 390 degrees F. Line a roasting pan with parchment paper.
2. Now, toss the carrots with the olive oil and arrange them on the prepared roasting pan.
3. Roast the carrots for about 50 minutes or until tender. Transfer the roasted carrots to the bowl of your food processor.

4. Add in the tahini, beans, garlic, lemon juice, soy sauce, salt, black pepper, paprika, and dill. Process until your dip is creamy and uniform.
5. Garnish with toasted pepitas and serve with dippers of choice.
6. Bon appétit!

SNACKS

Beans, Tomato & Corn Quesadillas

Ready in about: 15-30 minutes

Servings: 4

Per serve: Calories 197 Fats 6. 4g Carbs 30. 2g Protein 6. 6g

Ingredients:
- 2 tsps olive oil
- 2 small onions, chopped
- 1 medium red bell pepper, deseeded and chopped
- 2 (7 oz) can chopped tomatoes
- 2 (7 oz) can black beans, drained and rinsed
- 2 (7 oz) cans of sweet corn kernels, drained
- 8 whole-wheat tortillas
- 2 cups grated plant-based cheddar cheese

Directions:
1. Heat the olive oil in a medium skillet and sauté the onion and bell pepper until softened, 3 minutes.
2. Mix in the tomatoes, black beans, sweet corn, and cook until the tomatoes soften, 10 minutes. Season with salt and black pepper.
3. Heat another medium skillet over medium heat and lay in one tortilla. Spread a quarter of the tomato mixture on top, scatter a quarter of the plant cheese on the sauce, and cover with another

tortilla. Cook until the cheese melts. Flip and cook further for 2 minutes.

4. Transfer to a plate and make one more piece using the remaining ingredients.
5. Cut each tortilla set into quarters and serve immediately.
6. Enjoy!

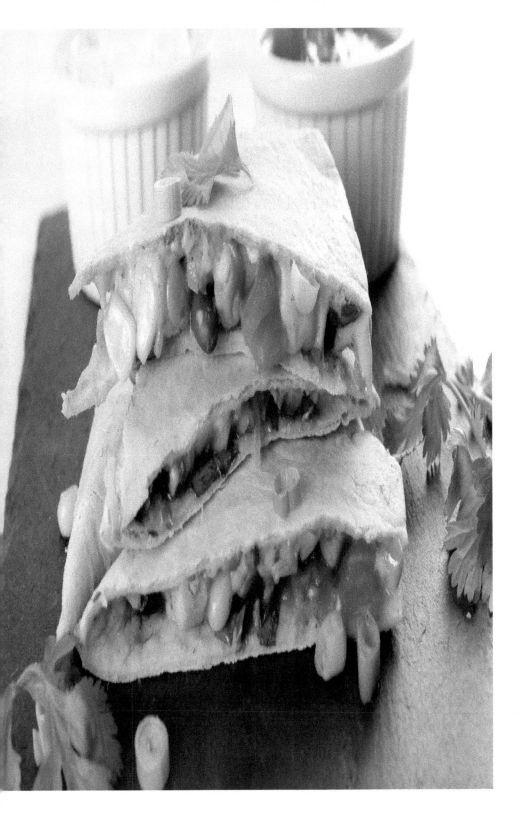

Buffalo Chickpea Wraps

Preparation Time: 20 minutes

Servings: 4

Per serving: Calories 254 Carbohydrates 39. 4 g Fats 6. 7 g Protein 9. 1 g

Ingredients:
- ½ cup plus 4 tablespoons hummus
- 4 tablespoons lemon juice
- 3 tablespoons maple syrup
- 2 to 4 tablespoons hot water
- 2 heads of Romaine lettuce, chopped
- 2 15-ounce can chickpeas, drained, rinsed, and patted dry
- 8 tablespoons hot sauce, divided
- 2 tablespoons olive or coconut oil
- ½ teaspoon garlic powder
- 2 pinches of sea salt
- 8 wheat tortillas
- ½ cup cherry tomatoes, diced
- ½ cup red onion, diced
- ½ of a ripe avocado, thinly sliced

Directions:
1. Mix the hummus with lemon juice and maple syrup in a large bowl. Use a whisk and add the hot

water, a little at a time, until it is thick but spreadable.

2. Add the Romaine lettuce and toss to coat. Set aside.
3. Pour the prepared chickpeas into another bowl. Add three tablespoons of the hot sauce, olive oil, garlic powder, and salt; toss to coat.
4. Heat a metal skillet (cast iron works the best) over medium heat and add the chickpea mixture. Sauté for three to five minutes and mash gently with a spoon.
5. Once the chickpea mixture is slightly dried out, remove it from the heat and add the rest of the hot sauce. Stir it in well and set aside.
6. Lay the tortillas on a clean, flat surface and spread a quarter cup of the buffalo chickpeas on top. Top with tomatoes, onion, and avocado (optional) and wrap.
7. Enjoy!!

Quinoa Cherry Tortilla Wraps

Preparation Time: 60 minutes

Servings: 8

Per serving: Calories 282 kcal Fats 6. 5g Carbs 48g Protein 8. 3g

Ingredients:

- 1 cup brown quinoa
- Salt and black pepper to taste
- 4 tsps olive oil
- 3 cups shredded carrots
- 5/2 cups fresh cherries, pitted and halved
- 8 scallions, chopped
- 4 tbsps plain vinegar
- 4 tbsps low-sodium soy sauce
- 2 tbsps pure maple syrup
- 8 (8-inch) tortilla wraps

Directions:

1. Cook the quinoa in 1 cup of slightly salted water in a medium pot over medium heat until tender and the water absorbs, 10 minutes. Fluff and set aside to warm.
2. Heat the olive oil in a medium skillet and sauté the carrots, cherries, and scallions. While cooking, in a small bowl, mix the vinegar, soy sauce, and maple syrup. Stir the mixture into the

vegetable mixture. Simmer for 5 minutes and turn the heat off.

3. Spread the tortillas on a flat surface, spoon the mixture at the center, fold the sides and ends to wrap in the filling.

4. Serve warm.

Balsamic Roasted Parsnip

Ready in about: 30 minutes

Servings: 12

Per serving: Calories: 174; Fat: 9.3g; Carbs: 22.2g; Protein: 1.4g

Ingredients

- 26 pounds parsnips, cut into sticks
- 1/2 cup olive oil
- 1/2 cup balsamic vinegar
- 2 teaspoons Dijon mustard
- 2 teaspoons fennel seeds
- Sea salt and ground black pepper, to taste
- 2 teaspoons Mediterranean spice mix

Directions

1. Toss all ingredients in a mixing bowl until the parsnips are well coated.
2. Roast the parsnip in the preheated oven at 400 degrees F for about 30 minutes, stirring halfway through the cooking time.
3. Serve at room temperature and enjoy!

Peanut Butter Date Bites

Ready in about: 5 minutes

Servings: 4

Per serving: Calories: 143; Fat: 3.9g; Carbs: 26.3g; Protein: 2.6g

Ingredients

- 16 fresh dates, pitted and cut into halves
- 16 teaspoons peanut butter
- 1/2 teaspoon ground cinnamon

Directions

1. Divide the peanut butter between the date halves.
2. Dust with cinnamon and serve immediately. Bon appétit

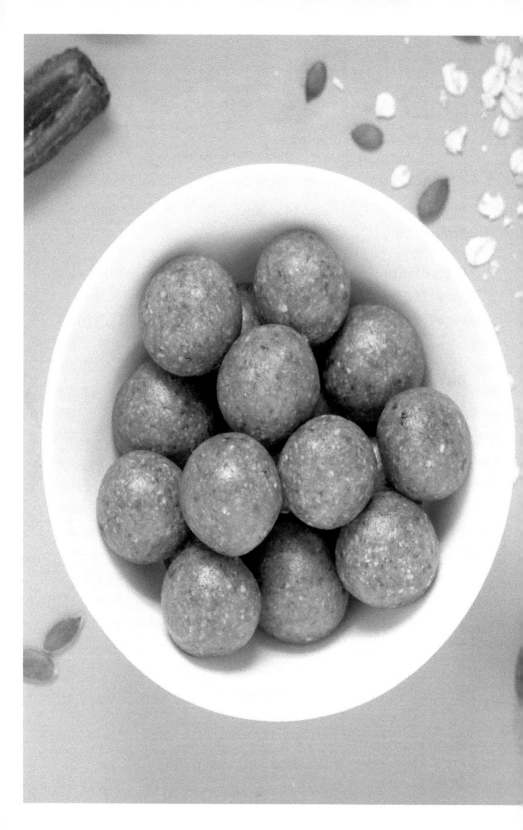

Roasted Cauliflower Dip

Ready in about: 30 minutes

Servings: 14

Per serving: Calories: 142; Fat: 12.5g; Carbs: 6.3g; Protein: 2.9g

Ingredients

- 2 pounds cauliflower florets
- 1/2 cup olive oil
- 8 tablespoons tahini
- 1 teaspoon paprika
- Sea salt and ground black pepper, to taste
- 4 tablespoons fresh lime juice
- 4 cloves garlic, minced

Directions

1. Start by preheating your oven to 420 degrees F. Toss the cauliflower florets with the olive oil and arrange them on a parchment-lined baking pan.
2. Bake for about 25 minutes or until tender.
3. Then, puree the cauliflower along with the remaining ingredients, adding cooking liquid as needed.
4. Drizzle with some extra olive oil, if desired. Bon appétit!

Chipotle Sweet Potato Fries

Ready in about: 45 minutes

Servings: 8

Per serving: Calories: 186; Fat: 7.1g; Carbs: 29.6g; Protein: 2.5g

Ingredients
- 8 medium sweet potatoes, peeled and cut into sticks
- 4 tablespoons peanut oil
- Sea salt and ground black pepper, to taste
- 2 teaspoons chipotle pepper powder
- 1/2 teaspoon ground allspice
- 2 teaspoons brown sugar
- 2 teaspoons dried rosemary

Directions
1. Toss the sweet potato fries with the remaining ingredients.
2. Bake your fries at 375 degrees F for about 45 minutes or until browned; make sure to stir the fries once or twice.
3. Serve with your favorite dipping sauce, if desired. Bon appétit!

Spiced Roasted Cauliflower

Ready in about: 25 minutes

Servings: 12

Per serving: Calories: 115; Fat: 9.3g; Carbs: 6.9g; Protein: 5.6g

Ingredients

- 3 pounds cauliflower florets
- 1/2 cup olive oil
- 8 tablespoons apple cider vinegar
- 4 cloves of garlic, pressed
- 2 teaspoons dried basil
- 2 teaspoons dried oregano
- Sea salt and ground black pepper, to taste

Directions

1. Begin by preheating your oven to 420 degrees F.
2. Toss the cauliflower florets with the remaining ingredients.
3. Arrange the cauliflower florets on a parchment-lined baking sheet. Bake the cauliflower florets in the preheated oven for about 25 minutes or until they are slightly charred.
4. Bon appétit!

Buttered Carrot Noodles with Kale

Ready in about: 15 minutes

Servings: 8

Ingredients

- 4 large carrots
- 1/2 cup vegetable broth
- 8 tbsps plant butter
- 2 garlic cloves, minced
- 2 cups chopped kale
- Salt and black pepper to taste

Directions

1. Peel the carrots with a slicer and run both through a spiralizer to form noodles.

2. Pour the vegetable broth into a saucepan and add the carrot noodles. Simmer (over low heat) the carrots for 3 minutes. Strain through a colander and set the vegetables aside.

3. Place a large skillet over medium heat and melt the plant butter. Add the garlic and sauté until softened and put in the kale; cook until wilted. Pour the carrots into the pan, season with salt and black pepper, and stir-fry for 3 to 4 minutes. Spoon the vegetables into a bowl and serve with pan-grilled tofu.

Curry Cauli Rice with Mushrooms

Ready in about: 15 minutes

Servings: 8

Ingredients

- 16 oz baby Bella mushrooms, stemmed and sliced
- 4 large heads of cauliflower
- 4 tbsps toasted sesame oil, divided
- 2 onions, chopped
- 6 garlic cloves, minced
- Salt and black pepper to taste
- 1 tsp curry powder
- 2 tsps freshly chopped parsley
- 4 scallions, thinly sliced

Directions

1. Use a knife to cut the entire cauliflower head into 6 pieces and transfer to a food processor. With the grater attachment, shred the cauliflower into a rice-like consistency.

2. Heat half of the sesame oil in a large skillet over medium heat, and then add the onion and mushrooms. Sauté for 5 minutes or until the mushrooms are soft.

3. Add the garlic and sauté for 2 minutes or until fragrant. Pour in the cauliflower and cook until

the rice has slightly softened for about 10 minutes.

4. Season with salt, black pepper, and curry powder; then, mix the ingredients to be well combined. After, turn the heat off and stir in the parsley and scallions. Dish the cauli rice into serving plates and serve warm.

Grilled Tofu Mayo Sandwiches

Ready in about: 15 minutes

Servings: 4

Ingredients

- ½ cup tofu mayonnaise
- 4 slices whole-grain bread
- ½ cucumber, sliced
- 1 cup lettuce, chopped
- 1 tomato, sliced
- 2 tsps olive oil, divided

Directions

1. Spread the vegan mayonnaise over a bread slice, top with the cucumber, lettuce, and tomato, and finish with the other slice. Heat the oil in a skillet over medium heat. Place the sandwich and grill for 3 minutes, then flip over and cook for a further 3 minutes. Cut the sandwich in half and serve.

2. Bon Appetit!

Baked Spicy Eggplant

Ready in about: 30 minutes | Servings: 8

Ingredients

- 4 large eggplants
- Salt and black pepper to taste
- 4 tbsps plant butter
- 2 tsps red chili flakes
- 8 oz raw ground almonds

Directions

1. Preheat oven to 400 F.

2. Cut off the head of the eggplants and slice the body into 2-inch rounds. Season with salt and black pepper and arrange on a parchment paper-lined baking sheet.

3. Drop thin slices of the plant butter on each eggplant slice, sprinkle with red chili flakes, and bake in the oven for 20 minutes.

4. Slide the baking sheet out and sprinkle with the almonds. Roast further for 5 minutes or until golden brown. Dish the eggplants and serve with arugula salad.

5. Enjoy!

CONCLUSION

There is a plethora of compelling reasons to make a positive difference and transition to a plant-based diet. A plant-based diet will increase your quality of life by providing you with more energy and stamina, assisting you in losing excess body weight, and perhaps even extending your time on this magnificent world. Too much energy and fossil fuels are lost in the process of obtaining meat and other animal products, shipping them over miles and miles of road, and refining them. You will also be bringing a genuine and important difference to the future of our planet Earth by making the transition.

By switching to rich plant-based meals, we can save the earth and also take care of ourselves.

Thank you for taking the time to read this.